THE HYDROGEN HEALTH REVOLUTION

A Comprehensive Guide to Therapeutic Applications in Adulthood

DR MORRIS HILLS

Table of Contents

INTRODUCTION

Hydrogen Medicine for Adults: Unveiling Scientific Insights and Mechanisms

In the realm of innovative healthcare, the concept of hydrogen medicine has emerged as a promising frontier, offering potential benefits for adult well-being. This introduction serves as a gateway into the exploration of scientific studies and mechanisms behind hydrogen therapy for adults, delving into a realm where molecular hydrogen becomes a beacon of hope in health interventions.

Unveiling Hydrogen Medicine

To embark on this journey, it is crucial to understand the essence of hydrogen medicine. At its core, hydrogen medicine involves the therapeutic use of molecular hydrogen (H2) to combat various health issues. Historically, hydrogen was often overlooked, considered a mere bystander in biological processes. However, recent scientific inquiries have illuminated its potential as a crucial player in maintaining health and mitigating diseases.

Historical Context

The historical backdrop of hydrogen medicine unveils its evolution from obscurity to a subject of intense scientific scrutiny. Traditionally dismissed as an inert gas with minimal biological relevance, hydrogen's therapeutic properties remained dormant. The narrative changed as pioneering researchers began to unravel its potential applications, leading to a paradigm shift in our understanding of molecular hydrogen.

Relevance in Contemporary Healthcare

As we navigate the landscape of modern healthcare, the relevance of hydrogen medicine becomes increasingly apparent. Amidst the complexities of adult health challenges, the potential of hydrogen therapy to intervene and complement existing medical practices takes center stage. The introduction explores how hydrogen medicine aligns with the demands of contemporary healthcare, offering a novel approach to address health issues that have persisted despite conventional treatments.

Capturing the Reader's Interest

To captivate the reader's interest, the introduction employs a narrative strategy that highlights the captivating story of an individual's journey through hydrogen medicine. This serves as a microcosm of the broader potential and impact of hydrogen therapy on adult health. By weaving a compelling narrative, the introduction aims to evoke curiosity, encouraging readers to delve deeper into the scientific studies and mechanisms that underpin this intriguing field.

Establishing Importance

The introduction establishes the importance of examining hydrogen medicine for adults by emphasizing its potential to fill gaps in conventional healthcare. By introducing the idea of hydrogen as a secret weapon against health challenges, it sets the stage for a comprehensive exploration of the scientific studies and mechanisms that validate its therapeutic efficacy. This section emphasizes that, in a world where existing systems may fall short, hydrogen medicine emerges as a beacon of hope.

Preview of Subsequent Sections

As a roadmap for the reader, the introduction concludes by offering a brief preview of the subsequent sections. These sections will delve into the scientific studies that substantiate the therapeutic claims of hydrogen medicine and explore the underlying mechanisms at play. By providing a glimpse into the forthcoming insights, the introduction encourages the reader to continue their exploration, armed with the understanding that hydrogen medicine holds the potential to reshape our approach to adult health.

In essence, this introduction serves as an invitation to unravel the mysteries of hydrogen medicine, beckoning readers to join the expedition into the scientific studies and mechanisms that illuminate its transformative power in the realm of adult healthcare.

Chapter 1: Unlocking the Basics of Hydrogen Medicine: A Comprehensive Exploration

In the ever-evolving landscape of medical science, hydrogen medicine has emerged as a captivating field with the potential to redefine healthcare paradigms. This in-depth exploration aims to dissect the basics of hydrogen medicine, shedding light on its origins, molecular intricacies, and foundational principles that underpin its therapeutic promise for adults.

Foundation of Molecular Hydrogen

At the heart of hydrogen medicine lies molecular hydrogen (H_2), a diatomic molecule composed of two hydrogen atoms. Once relegated to the sidelines as an inert gas, molecular hydrogen has now ascended to a position of prominence in medical research. Understanding its basic properties, such as its ability to permeate cellular barriers and act as a selective antioxidant, sets the stage for comprehending the transformative potential it holds within the realm of healthcare.

Antioxidant Properties

Delving into the basics requires an exploration of hydrogen's remarkable antioxidant properties. Unlike traditional antioxidants, molecular hydrogen demonstrates selectivity in neutralizing harmful reactive oxygen species (ROS) while sparing essential signaling molecules. This section elucidates how hydrogen's unique antioxidant mechanisms contribute to cellular balance, potentially mitigating oxidative stress implicated in various health conditions.

Cellular Signaling and Anti-Inflammatory Effects

The basics extend beyond mere antioxidant prowess, encompassing the profound impact of hydrogen on cellular signaling pathways. Hydrogen exerts modulatory effects on signaling molecules, influencing vital cellular processes. By dissecting these mechanisms, we gain insight into how hydrogen may exert anti-inflammatory effects, a facet crucial for addressing conditions where chronic inflammation plays a central role.

Hydrogen in Action: Metabolism and Energy Production

A foundational understanding of hydrogen medicine involves unraveling its influence on metabolic processes and energy production. Hydrogen's interaction with mitochondria, the cellular powerhouses, emerges as a key aspect. Exploring how hydrogen may enhance mitochondrial function sheds light on its potential implications for adult health, particularly in contexts where energy imbalance contributes to pathologies.

Gut Microbiota: A Nexus of Health

Venturing into the basics unveils an intriguing connection between hydrogen and gut microbiota. Hydrogen serves as a modulator of the microbial landscape, impacting the delicate balance within the digestive system. This section elucidates how hydrogen's influence on gut microbiota may contribute to overall well-being, presenting a novel dimension in our understanding of its therapeutic potential.

Practical Applications in Adult Health

The basics of hydrogen medicine extend into practical applications, providing a bridge between molecular intricacies and real-world impact. This section explores specific health conditions where hydrogen therapy shows promise for adults. From neurodegenerative disorders to cardiovascular health, the basics serve as a foundation for comprehending the diverse avenues where hydrogen medicine may offer therapeutic benefits.

Safety Considerations and Dosage Guidelines

An integral part of the basics involves addressing safety considerations and establishing dosage guidelines. Understanding the parameters that ensure the safe administration of hydrogen therapy is paramount for its integration into mainstream healthcare. This section navigates through existing research and recommendations, offering insights into the responsible application of hydrogen medicine for adult populations.

Future Directions and Unanswered Questions

Concluding the exploration of the basics, it is essential to peer into the future of hydrogen medicine. Unanswered questions and potential avenues for research beckon, inviting scientists and healthcare practitioners to delve deeper. This section sparks curiosity about the evolving nature of hydrogen medicine and the exciting possibilities that lie ahead.

In essence, this comprehensive journey through the basics of hydrogen medicine aims to equip readers with a nuanced understanding of its foundational elements. From molecular intricacies to practical applications, this exploration lays the groundwork for unraveling the mysteries that make hydrogen medicine a compelling frontier in the pursuit of adult health and well-being.

Chapter 2: Unveiling the Intricacies: Mechanisms of Hydrogen Therapy Explored

As the landscape of medical science continues to evolve, the exploration of innovative therapeutic modalities gains momentum. Among these, hydrogen therapy has emerged as a captivating subject, harnessing the potential of molecular hydrogen (H2) to foster health and well-being. This in-depth analysis aims to dissect the mechanisms that underpin hydrogen therapy, unraveling the complex interplay between molecular hydrogen and biological systems.

Molecular Hydrogen: A Cellular Penetrator

At the core of hydrogen therapy lies the unique ability of molecular hydrogen to traverse cellular barriers with remarkable ease. Unlike many therapeutic agents, H2's small size and non-polar nature enable it to access cellular compartments, including the nucleus and mitochondria. This section delves into the implications of this exceptional feature, highlighting how H2's cellular penetrative ability sets the stage for its multifaceted therapeutic effects.

Selective Antioxidant Properties

Hydrogen's role as a selective antioxidant stands as a hallmark of its therapeutic potential. In contrast to conventional antioxidants, which may neutralize both harmful reactive oxygen species (ROS) and essential signaling molecules, molecular hydrogen exhibits a discriminative capacity. This segment elucidates the mechanisms through which H2 selectively targets and neutralizes detrimental ROS, preserving crucial signaling pathways that regulate cellular functions.

Modulation of Cellular Signaling

Beyond its antioxidant prowess, hydrogen therapy extends its influence into the realm of cellular signaling. This section unravels the intricate mechanisms through which H2 modulates signaling pathways, impacting fundamental cellular processes. By elucidating these signaling cascades, a deeper understanding emerges of how hydrogen therapy may exert regulatory effects on inflammation, apoptosis, and other pathways implicated in various health conditions.

Anti-Inflammatory Pathways

Chronic inflammation constitutes a common denominator in diverse pathological states. Hydrogen therapy emerges as a modulator of inflammatory responses, showcasing its potential as an anti-inflammatory agent.

Investigating the specific pathways through which molecular hydrogen interferes with inflammatory cascades provides insights into its role in managing conditions where inflammation plays a pivotal role, from neurodegenerative disorders to autoimmune conditions.

Metabolic Influences and Energy Dynamics

Hydrogen's impact on cellular metabolism and energy production adds another layer to its multifaceted mechanisms. Particularly relevant in conditions characterized by metabolic dysregulation, this segment explores how H2 interacts with mitochondria, the cellular powerhouses. Unraveling the nuances of hydrogen's influence on metabolic pathways sheds light on its potential implications for conditions such as metabolic syndrome and related disorders.

Gut Microbiota: A Mediator of Health

The intricate relationship between hydrogen therapy and gut microbiota unfolds as a fascinating aspect of its mechanisms. H2's influence on the microbial community within the digestive system holds implications for overall health. This section navigates through the dynamic interplay between hydrogen and gut microbiota, exploring how this interaction contributes to the therapeutic effects observed in various physiological and pathological contexts.

Neuroprotective Pathways

The neuroprotective potential of hydrogen therapy takes center stage in the context of neurological disorders. From neurodegenerative conditions to acute brain injuries, molecular hydrogen demonstrates promising effects. This segment dissects the mechanisms underlying hydrogen's neuroprotective actions, shedding light on how it may safeguard neuronal integrity and function.

Cardiovascular Implications

Exploring the cardiovascular implications of hydrogen therapy unveils a spectrum of mechanisms that impact heart health. From antioxidant effects that protect against oxidative stress in vascular tissues to the modulation of blood pressure, this section unravels the cardiovascular intricacies of H2. Understanding these mechanisms paves the way for considering hydrogen therapy as a complementary approach in cardiovascular care.

Safety Considerations and Dosage Optimization

Ensuring the safe and effective application of hydrogen therapy necessitates a thorough examination of safety considerations and optimal dosage guidelines. This segment synthesizes existing research and recommendations, providing a comprehensive guide for healthcare practitioners and researchers. Addressing concerns related to hydrogen concentration, delivery methods, and potential side effects contributes to the responsible integration of hydrogen therapy into clinical practice.

Future Horizons: Unanswered Questions and Promising Avenues

As we delve into the mechanisms of hydrogen therapy, it becomes apparent that many questions remain unanswered. This section serves as a bridge to the future, inviting exploration into yet undiscovered facets of H2's mechanisms. From unraveling novel pathways to optimizing delivery modalities, the evolving nature of hydrogen therapy beckons researchers to embark on a journey of discovery.

In essence, this comprehensive exploration of the mechanisms of hydrogen therapy endeavors to unravel the intricacies that render molecular hydrogen a compelling agent in the pursuit of health and well-being. From its cellular penetrative abilities to the modulation of intricate pathways, hydrogen therapy stands at the forefront of innovative approaches, inviting continued research and application in diverse medical contexts.

Chapter 4: Hydrogen Medicine Unveiled: A Historical Odyssey

As we venture into the realms of hydrogen medicine, a journey through its historical tapestry reveals a narrative woven with scientific curiosity, discovery, and the evolution of medical understanding. The historical perspective of hydrogen medicine in adults takes us back to the inception of this intriguing field and traces its trajectory through key milestones, scientific breakthroughs, and the gradual assimilation of hydrogen's therapeutic potential into medical discourse.

Ancient Notions and Elemental Beginnings

While the formalization of hydrogen medicine as a distinct field occurred in modern times, historical echoes of hydrogen's significance reverberate through ancient wisdom. Early civilizations, albeit unknowingly, interacted with hydrogen in its elemental form. From the alchemists' quest for the philosopher's stone to the elemental philosophers of ancient Greece contemplating the building blocks of matter, hydrogen's subtle presence permeated early scientific thought.

Hydrogen's Discovery and Early Chemical Exploration

The 18th century marked a pivotal period with the discovery and isolation of hydrogen by Henry Cavendish. This gaseous element, with its lightness and flammability, intrigued scientists and laid the groundwork for understanding its chemical properties. As hydrogen found its place in the periodic table, a new chapter in chemistry unfolded, setting the stage for later explorations into its therapeutic potential.

Hydrogen Inhalation Therapy: Early 20th Century

The early 20th century witnessed the first glimpses of hydrogen's medicinal applications, primarily through inhalation therapy. Medical practitioners explored the inhalation of hydrogen gas for various respiratory conditions, inspired by the perceived benefits of breathing hydrogen-rich air. While these early attempts lacked the rigorous scientific scrutiny of contemporary research, they laid the groundwork for future investigations into the physiological effects of molecular hydrogen.

The Rise of Hydrogen-Rich Water

Advancements in hydrogen medicine gained momentum in the latter half of the 20th century, with a notable shift towards exploring the benefits of hydrogen-rich water. Japanese researchers played a pivotal role in this era, recognizing the potential health-promoting properties of water infused with molecular hydrogen. The emergence of electrolysis devices capable of producing hydrogen-rich water fueled a new wave of scientific interest and inquiry.

Milestones in Scientific Validation

The turn of the 21st century ushered in a surge of scientific studies focused on elucidating the mechanisms and therapeutic potential of hydrogen. Notable milestones include the landmark 2007 publication in Nature Medicine, which demonstrated the antioxidant properties of hydrogen by selectively reducing hydroxyl radicals.

Subsequent studies expanded the scope, exploring hydrogen's impact on inflammation, metabolism, and various disease models.

Diverse Applications in Adult Health

Hydrogen medicine's historical evolution mirrors the broadening scope of its applications in adult health. From neurological disorders to cardiovascular conditions, research has explored hydrogen's potential benefits across diverse medical landscapes. Neuroprotective effects, cardiovascular implications, and anti-inflammatory properties have emerged as key areas of interest, fostering the integration of hydrogen therapy into the multifaceted realm of adult healthcare.

The Global Landscape of Hydrogen Research

The historical journey of hydrogen medicine extends globally, with researchers and healthcare practitioners around the world contributing to its expansion. Collaborative efforts have led to a nuanced understanding of hydrogen's mechanisms and its potential in addressing a spectrum of health challenges. The collective endeavor to unravel the intricacies of hydrogen's interactions with the human body has transformed it from a historical curiosity to a subject of contemporary scientific exploration.

Challenges and Uncharted Territories

As hydrogen medicine unfolds its historical narrative, it is essential to acknowledge the challenges and uncharted territories that accompany this evolving field. Questions regarding optimal dosages, long-term effects, and personalized applications linger, beckoning researchers to delve deeper into the complexities of hydrogen's interactions with the human physiology.

In conclusion, the historical perspective of hydrogen medicine in adults unveils a captivating journey from ancient musings to modern scientific rigor. From elemental beginnings to the global landscape of contemporary research, hydrogen's therapeutic odyssey continues to captivate the scientific community. As we stand at the crossroads of historical insights and future possibilities, hydrogen medicine beckons with the promise of unlocking new dimensions in the pursuit of human health and well-being.

Chapter 5: Exploring Molecular Hydrogen: Properties and Forms

Molecular hydrogen, a diatomic molecule consisting of two hydrogen atoms, H2, has emerged as a fascinating subject of scientific inquiry and therapeutic exploration. Beyond its ubiquitous presence in the cosmos, molecular hydrogen's unique properties and diverse forms captivate researchers, promising a spectrum of applications ranging from medicine to energy. This deep dive into the properties and forms of molecular hydrogen unveils the molecular intricacies that render it a compelling player in various scientific arenas.

Molecular Ballet: Properties of Molecular Hydrogen

1. Diatomic Dance: Structure and Stability
At its core, molecular hydrogen is a diatomic molecule, meaning it consists of two hydrogen atoms covalently bonded. This simple yet elegant structure conceals a stability that belies its explosive reputation in its elemental form. The H2 molecule's symmetrical arrangement contributes to its inertness under standard conditions, making it a stable and non-reactive entity.

2. The Lightness Quotient: Physical Properties
One of molecular hydrogen's defining characteristics is its remarkable lightness. This attribute manifests in its low molecular weight, enabling it to diffuse rapidly through various mediums, including cellular structures. This physical property underlies its potential as a therapeutic agent,

facilitating its swift penetration into biological tissues.

3. Hydrogen's Therapeutic Arsenal: Antioxidant Prowess

A key facet of molecular hydrogen's therapeutic allure lies in its role as a selective antioxidant. Unlike traditional antioxidants, hydrogen selectively targets and neutralizes highly reactive and harmful free radicals, particularly the hydroxyl radical. This unique antioxidant capacity arises from hydrogen's ability to undergo redox reactions, contributing to cellular homeostasis and mitigating oxidative stress.

4. Gas with a Memory: Molecular Memory Effects

Molecular hydrogen exhibits intriguing memory effects, retaining information about its exposure conditions. This phenomenon, known as "memory of water" or "hydrogen memory," raises questions about the potential long-term effects and implications of hydrogen-rich environments. Researchers delve into this phenomenon, exploring its relevance in therapeutic applications and its broader implications for understanding molecular interactions.

Dynamic Forms: Hydrogen's Multifaceted Manifestations

1. Hydrogen-Rich Water: Liquid Emissary of Hydrogen

Hydrogen-rich water represents a tangible and accessible form of molecular hydrogen. Produced through various methods, such as electrolysis or dissolving hydrogen-producing tablets, this liquid form encapsulates molecular hydrogen for convenient consumption. Its popularity in hydrogen medicine stems from its simplicity and the ease with which it integrates into daily hydration practices.

2. Hydrogen Gas Inhalation: Breath of Therapeutic Air

Inhalation of hydrogen gas stands as a direct route to harnessing its therapeutic potential. The respiratory system serves as a gateway for molecular hydrogen to enter circulation, facilitating its distribution to target tissues. This form of administration has garnered attention for its potential in addressing respiratory conditions and promoting systemic effects.

3. Hydrogen-Embedded Materials: Solid Foundations

Innovations in materials science have led to the development of hydrogen-embedded materials, wherein hydrogen is absorbed or bonded to a solid matrix. These materials offer a sustained release of molecular hydrogen, presenting opportunities for controlled and prolonged therapeutic delivery. From hydrogen-infused ceramics to metal hydrides, these solid forms open avenues for diverse applications.

4. Hydrogen-Generating Devices:
Technological Allies
Advancements in technology have given rise to portable hydrogen-generating devices, allowing on-demand production of molecular hydrogen. These devices often utilize chemical reactions or electrolysis to liberate hydrogen gas for immediate use. Their portability and convenience position them as practical tools for individuals seeking real-time access to molecular hydrogen.

Navigating the Future: Unveiling Potential Applications

1. Therapeutic Frontiers: Clinical and Preventive Applications
As our understanding of molecular hydrogen deepens, its potential applications in clinical and preventive medicine continue to expand. From neurological disorders and cardiovascular health to anti-aging

interventions, researchers explore the therapeutic frontiers that molecular hydrogen may traverse. Clinical trials and studies illuminate the path, shedding light on its efficacy and safety in diverse medical contexts.

2. Energy Landscapes: Hydrogen as a Sustainable Resource
Beyond medicine, molecular hydrogen plays a pivotal role in the realm of sustainable energy. As a clean and efficient fuel, hydrogen holds promise in powering fuel cells, driving vehicles, and contributing to a renewable energy landscape. Research endeavors delve into harnessing hydrogen's energy potential while addressing challenges related to production, storage, and infrastructure.

Conclusion: Molecular Hydrogen's Enigmatic Charm

In conclusion, the exploration of molecular hydrogen's properties and forms unravels a tapestry of scientific marvels and therapeutic potential. From the diatomic ballet of its molecular structure to the diverse manifestations encapsulated in hydrogen-rich water, inhalation, solid materials, and cutting-edge devices, molecular hydrogen captivates with its multifaceted nature. As researchers navigate the uncharted territories of its applications, the enigmatic charm of molecular hydrogen persists, beckoning us toward a future where its benefits may shape both healthcare and sustainable energy landscapes.

Chapter 6: Unraveling the Intricacies: The Antioxidant Symphony in Adult Health

In the intricate dance of human biology, antioxidants emerge as unsung heroes, wielding protective prowess against the relentless onslaught of oxidative stress. As adults traverse the journey of life, the delicate equilibrium between oxidants and antioxidants becomes a linchpin for health and well-being. This exploration delves into the multifaceted world of antioxidants, unraveling their roles, mechanisms, and impact on adult health.

I. The Oxidative Tightrope: Understanding Oxidative Stress

1. Oxidative Stress Unveiled

At the heart of antioxidant function lies the concept of oxidative stress – a delicate imbalance between reactive oxygen species (ROS) and the body's antioxidant defenses. ROS, generated during normal metabolic processes or in response to external factors, pose a dual nature: essential signaling molecules in moderation, yet destructive forces when their levels spiral out of control. Oxidative stress serves as a linchpin in aging, chronic diseases, and various health challenges.

2. Culprits of Chaos: Sources of Oxidative Stress

Unraveling the sources of oxidative stress illuminates the myriad challenges adults face. From environmental pollutants and UV radiation to internal factors like inflammation and mitochondrial dysfunction, the origins of ROS are diverse and omnipresent. Understanding these sources sets the stage for comprehending the significance of antioxidants in maintaining a delicate balance.

II. Antioxidant Arsenal: Guardians of Cellular Harmony

1. Enzymatic Guardians: Superoxide Dismutase, Catalase, and Glutathione

Within the cellular realm, a triad of enzymatic guardians orchestrates the defense against ROS. Superoxide dismutase, catalase, and glutathione peroxidase form a formidable alliance, neutralizing superoxide anions, hydrogen peroxide, and lipid peroxides. The intricate interplay of these enzymes ensures that the cellular orchestra remains in harmony, thwarting the potential havoc wreaked by unchecked ROS.

2. Vitamin Avengers: A, C, and E

The vitamin triumvirate – A, C, and E – don the mantle of antioxidants, each contributing unique strengths to the defense against oxidative stress. Vitamin A's role in maintaining vision and skin health intertwines with its antioxidant properties.

Vitamin C, a water-soluble powerhouse, regenerates other antioxidants and shields cellular components. Meanwhile, vitamin E, a lipid-soluble protector, guards cell membranes from oxidation. Together, these vitamins form a frontline defense, scavenging free radicals and mitigating oxidative damage.

3. Polyphenols: Nature's Emissaries

Embarking on a journey through plant-derived compounds, polyphenols emerge as nature's emissaries in the battle against oxidative stress. Found in fruits, vegetables, tea, and red wine, polyphenols exhibit a spectrum of antioxidant activities. Flavonoids, anthocyanins, and resveratrol stand out among these, showcasing their ability to modulate cellular signaling, combat inflammation, and bolster antioxidant defenses.

III. Antioxidants in Action: Impact on Adult Health

1. Cardiovascular Symphony: Safeguarding the Heart

The cardiovascular system stands as a poignant testament to the impact of antioxidants on adult health. Oxidative stress plays a pivotal role in atherosclerosis and heart diseases. Antioxidants, by mitigating inflammation and lipid peroxidation, contribute to arterial health and the prevention of cardiovascular events. The interplay between antioxidants and endothelial function becomes a crucial chapter in this cardiovascular symphony.

2. Neural Harmony: Antioxidants and Brain Health

Within the intricate folds of the brain, antioxidants orchestrate a delicate dance to safeguard neural harmony. The aging brain faces challenges from oxidative stress, contributing to neurodegenerative diseases. Antioxidants, with their ability to cross the blood-brain barrier, exert neuroprotective effects, potentially slowing cognitive decline and promoting optimal brain function in adults.

3. Cellular Rejuvenation: Antioxidants and Aging

As the chronological clock ticks, the cellular landscape undergoes transformations influenced by oxidative stress. Antioxidants, by virtue of their scavenging abilities and influence on cellular signaling pathways, contribute to cellular rejuvenation. The impact on skin health, joint function, and overall vitality becomes evident as antioxidants navigate the complex terrain of aging, offering a semblance of resilience against time's relentless march.

IV. Lifestyle Choices: Nurturing the Antioxidant Symphony

1. Nutritional Maestro: Dietary Habits and Antioxidant Intake

The nutritional maestro conducts a symphony of health through dietary habits. A diet rich in fruits, vegetables, nuts, and whole grains provides a plethora of antioxidants, fortifying the body's defenses. Exploring the nuances of antioxidant-rich foods becomes paramount in crafting a dietary repertoire that fosters resilience against oxidative stress.

2. Exercise as a Crescendo: Physical Activity and Antioxidant Defense

The crescendo of physical activity reverberates through the antioxidant landscape. Regular exercise enhances endogenous antioxidant defenses, promoting a robust shield against oxidative stress. Unraveling the intricacies of exercise-induced adaptations illuminates the role of physical activity as a lifestyle choice that complements the antioxidant symphony.

V. Challenges and Frontiers: Navigating the Unknown

1. Antioxidants in Disease: Therapeutic Potential and Complexities

Delving into the therapeutic potential of antioxidants unveils a complex landscape. While studies suggest promising outcomes in various diseases, the intricacies of dosage, timing, and individual variations pose challenges. Navigating the unknown involves unraveling the context-dependent nature of antioxidant interventions, opening avenues for precision medicine in the realm of antioxidants.

2. Beyond the Horizon: Antioxidants in Aging Research

The quest to unlock the secrets of aging beckons researchers beyond the horizon of conventional wisdom. Antioxidants, with their implications for cellular senescence and longevity, become focal points in aging research. Exploring the frontiers of mitochondrial health, telomere dynamics, and epigenetic modulation unveils potential avenues for extending the healthspan of adults.

Conclusion: The Ever-Evolving Symphony of Antioxidants

In conclusion, the antioxidant symphony in adult health unfolds as a multifaceted composition, weaving together enzymatic defenders, vitamin avengers, and nature's emissaries in polyphenols. From cardiovascular safeguards to neural harmonies and cellular rejuvenation, antioxidants stand as integral players in the pursuit of optimal health. Nurturing this symphony through lifestyle choices, dietary habits, and ongoing research into therapeutic frontiers invites individuals to actively participate in the ever-evolving narrative of antioxidant-driven well-being. As adults navigate the complexities of health, the antioxidant symphony remains a dynamic force, harmonizing the delicate balance between oxidative stress and resilient vitality.

Unraveling the Tapestry: Anti-Inflammatory Effects on Adult Physiology

In the intricate tapestry of adult physiology, the role of inflammation emerges as a double-edged sword. While acute inflammation is a fundamental defense mechanism, chronic inflammation becomes a silent assailant, contributing to a myriad of health challenges. This exploration delves into the profound impact of anti-inflammatory mechanisms on adult physiology, shedding light on the intricate pathways, molecular players, and the far-reaching consequences of modulating inflammation.

I. Inflammation Unveiled: The Physiological Dynamics

1. The Yin and Yang of Inflammation

At its core, inflammation represents a complex orchestration of molecular and cellular events designed to protect the body from harmful stimuli. The dichotomy of inflammation unfolds as a dynamic interplay between pro-inflammatory and anti-inflammatory signals. Acute inflammation serves as a swift, localized response, promoting healing and pathogen clearance. However, when inflammation persists or becomes dysregulated, the stage is set for chronic health conditions.

2. Cellular Architects: Immune System Dynamics

The immune system emerges as the architectural force behind inflammation, with immune cells acting as sentinels and effectors. Neutrophils, macrophages, and lymphocytes navigate the intricate landscape, releasing cytokines, chemokines, and other signaling molecules. This cellular symphony orchestrates the inflammatory cascade, culminating in tissue repair or, in chronic scenarios, tissue damage.

II. Molecular Players: Navigating the Inflammatory Landscape

1. Cytokine Symphony: Balancing Act of Signaling Molecules

Central to the inflammatory narrative, cytokines conduct a symphony of signaling, exerting both pro- and anti-inflammatory effects. Tumor necrosis factor-alpha (TNF-α), interleukins (IL), and transforming growth factor-beta (TGF-β) are key players in this intricate dance. Understanding the delicate balance of cytokine signaling provides insights into the modulation of inflammation and its impact on adult physiology.

2. NF-κB Pathway: Maestro of Inflammatory Transcription

Unraveling the NF-κB pathway unveils the maestro orchestrating the transcription of inflammatory genes. As a central regulator, NF-κB bridges extracellular signals to the nucleus, influencing the expression of pro-inflammatory mediators. The modulation of this pathway becomes a focal point in interventions aimed at curbing chronic inflammation and preserving adult physiological equilibrium.

III. Anti-Inflammatory Arsenal: Nature's Remedies

1. Omega-3 Fatty Acids: Nourishing Inflammatory Resolution

Embarking on a journey through dietary interventions, omega-3 fatty acids emerge as potent modulators of inflammation. Eicosapentaenoic acid (EPA) and docosahexaenoic acid (DHA) navigate cellular membranes, influencing the production of pro-resolving lipid mediators. The anti-inflammatory prowess of omega-3 fatty acids extends to diverse physiological domains, from cardiovascular health to neural well-being.

2. Polyphenolic Guardians: Quenching the Flames of Inflammation

Nature's pharmacy unfolds in the realm of polyphenols, showcasing their anti-inflammatory properties. Flavonoids, curcumin, and resveratrol stand as guardians, quenching the flames of inflammation through diverse molecular mechanisms. The intricate dance between polyphenols and inflammatory pathways becomes a testament to the potential of plant-derived compounds in modulating adult physiology.

IV. Impact on Adult Health: A Symphony of Resilience

1. Cardiovascular Harmony: Anti-Inflammatory Shields

Chronic inflammation intricately weaves its threads into the fabric of cardiovascular health. Anti-inflammatory interventions exhibit a symphony of resilience, safeguarding against atherosclerosis, endothelial dysfunction, and hypertension. The modulation of inflammatory markers becomes a key chapter in the narrative of cardiovascular harmony, showcasing the potential for targeted interventions.

2. Joint Wellness: Mitigating Inflammatory Arthritides

In the realm of musculoskeletal health, the impact of anti-inflammatory strategies extends to joints and connective tissues. Rheumatoid arthritis, osteoarthritis, and other inflammatory arthritides find themselves under the influence of interventions aimed at dampening inflammatory cascades. The preservation of joint wellness becomes a testament to the far-reaching effects of mitigating chronic inflammation.

3. Cognitive Resilience: Anti-Inflammatory Shields for the Brain

The intricate folds of the brain bear witness to the consequences of chronic inflammation, with implications for neurodegenerative diseases. Anti-inflammatory agents, traversing the blood-brain barrier, exhibit neuroprotective effects. The narrative of cognitive resilience unfolds as researchers explore the potential of anti-inflammatory interventions in mitigating cognitive decline and promoting brain health in adults.

V. Lifestyle Strategies: Cultivating Anti-Inflammatory Resilience

1. Dietary Symphony: Nourishing Inflammatory Balance

The dietary symphony echoes through the corridors of anti-inflammatory resilience. Embracing a diet rich in fruits, vegetables, fatty fish, and whole grains becomes a cornerstone in cultivating an environment of inflammatory balance. Unveiling the nuances of the anti-inflammatory diet empowers adults to make informed choices that resonate with physiological well-being.

2. Stress Management: Orchestrating Hormonal Equilibrium

Stress, a silent contributor to inflammation, finds its place in the narrative of anti-inflammatory resilience. Hormonal imbalances induced by chronic stress amplify inflammatory responses. Stress management strategies, from mindfulness to exercise, emerge as essential tools in orchestrating hormonal equilibrium and mitigating the inflammatory toll on adult physiology.

VI. Challenges and Frontiers: Navigating Complexity

1. Precision Medicine in Inflammation: Tailoring Interventions

The landscape of inflammation encompasses intricate individual variations, necessitating a precision medicine approach. Unraveling the complexities of genetic predispositions, microbiome influences, and personalized responses to anti-inflammatory interventions becomes a frontier in navigating the diverse terrain of adult physiology. Tailoring interventions to individual profiles holds the key to optimizing outcomes in the realm of inflammation.

2. Beyond Symptomatic Relief: Unraveling Root Causes

While anti-inflammatory strategies offer symptomatic relief, unraveling the root causes of chronic inflammation becomes paramount. Exploring the interplay between lifestyle factors, environmental influences, and genetic predispositions unveils avenues for comprehensive approaches to address the underlying drivers of inflammation. The quest for understanding the intricate tapestry of inflammation continues, prompting a holistic perspective on adult health.

Conclusion: Orchestrating Balance in Adult Physiology

In conclusion, the symphony of anti-inflammatory effects on adult physiology unfolds as a dynamic composition, with molecular players, dietary interventions, and lifestyle strategies contributing to a narrative of resilience.

From cardiovascular harmony to cognitive well-being, the impact of dampening chronic inflammation resonates across diverse physiological domains. As adults navigate the complexities of health, the orchestration of balance in inflammation becomes a pivotal theme, inviting individuals to actively participate in the ongoing narrative of physiological well-being.

Chapter 8: Cellular Signaling and Hydrogen Medicine

Cellular signaling and hydrogen medicine are fascinating fields that delve into the intricate mechanisms governing communication within cells and explore the potential therapeutic applications of molecular hydrogen. Let's embark on an exploration of these two areas.

Cellular Signaling:

Cellular signaling, also known as cell signaling or cell communication, is a complex network of processes that enable cells to perceive and respond to their environment. This intricate system ensures coordination and homeostasis in multicellular organisms. Cellular signaling involves the transmission of signals, often in the form of molecules, which bind to specific receptors on the cell surface or within the cell, triggering a cascade of events.

Types of Cellular Signaling:

1. **Autocrine Signaling:** In this type of signaling, cells release signaling molecules that bind to receptors on their own surface, influencing their own activity.

2. **Paracrine Signaling:** Signaling molecules are released into the extracellular fluid, affecting nearby cells. This is common in the immune system and during development.

3. **Endocrine Signaling:** Hormones, produced by specialized glands, travel through the bloodstream to target cells in distant parts of the body. This type of signaling is crucial for maintaining overall homeostasis.

4. Direct Cell-to-Cell Signaling: In some cases, cells can communicate directly through structures like gap junctions or plasmodesmata, allowing the passage of ions and small molecules between adjacent cells.

Signal Transduction Pathway:

When a signaling molecule binds to its receptor, it initiates a series of events known as a *signal transduction pathway*. This cascade often involves various proteins, enzymes, and second messengers, ultimately leading to a cellular response. The response can range from changes in gene expression to alterations in cell metabolism or movement.

Hydrogen Medicine:

Hydrogen medicine, or molecular hydrogen therapy, is an emerging field that explores the potential health benefits of molecular hydrogen (H2) gas. Initially considered inert, hydrogen has gained attention for its antioxidant and anti-inflammatory properties.

Mechanisms of Hydrogen Medicine:

1. **Antioxidant Effects:** Molecular hydrogen acts as a selective antioxidant, neutralizing harmful reactive oxygen species (ROS) without affecting essential signaling molecules like hydrogen peroxide.

2. **Anti-Inflammatory Properties:** Hydrogen has demonstrated anti-inflammatory effects by modulating various cellular pathways and reducing the production of pro-inflammatory cytokines.

3. **Cellular Energy Regulation:** H2 may influence cellular energy production by interacting with mitochondria and enhancing ATP (adenosine triphosphate) synthesis.

Methods of Hydrogen Administration:

1. **Hydrogen-Enriched Water:** Drinking water infused with molecular hydrogen is a simple and widely used method.

2. **Hydrogen Inhalation:** Inhaling hydrogen gas allows for rapid absorption into the bloodstream, reaching tissues and cells throughout the body.

3. **Hydrogen-Rich Saline:** Hydrogen dissolved in saline solutions can be administered intravenously, providing a more direct route to systemic circulation.

Cellular Signaling and Hydrogen Medicine Integration:

There's a growing interest in understanding how hydrogen medicine intersects with cellular signaling. Hydrogen's potential to modulate signaling pathways makes it an intriguing candidate for influencing cellular responses.

1. **Oxidative Stress and Signaling:** The antioxidant properties of hydrogen may impact cellular signaling pathways that are sensitive to oxidative stress. By scavenging ROS, hydrogen could indirectly influence signal transduction.

2. **Inflammation and Signal Transduction:** Hydrogen's anti-inflammatory effects may intersect with signaling pathways related to immune response and inflammation. This could have implications for conditions characterized by chronic inflammation.

3. **Mitochondrial Function and Cellular Signaling:** As hydrogen interacts with mitochondria, its influence on cellular energy production might have downstream effects on signaling pathways related to metabolism and cell survival.

4. Cellular Redox Balance: The delicate balance between oxidants and antioxidants is crucial for cellular function. Hydrogen's ability to maintain this balance may impact redox-sensitive signaling pathways.

Research and Clinical Implications:

Research in the intersection of cellular signaling and hydrogen medicine is still in its early stages, but initial findings suggest promising therapeutic potential. Clinical trials are underway to investigate the efficacy of hydrogen therapy in various medical conditions, including neurodegenerative disorders, cardiovascular diseases, and inflammatory conditions.

In summary, cellular signaling orchestrates the intricate dance of communication within our bodies, ensuring proper responses to internal and external stimuli. Hydrogen medicine, with its antioxidant and anti-inflammatory properties, offers a unique avenue for potential therapeutic interventions. As research progresses, the integration of these fields may uncover novel strategies for addressing a myriad of health conditions through the modulation of cellular signaling pathways.

Chapter 9: Impact on Mitochondrial Function in Adults: Unveiling the Core of Cellular Energy Dynamics

Mitochondria, often referred to as the powerhouse of the cell, play a pivotal role in cellular energy production and various metabolic processes. Understanding the impact on mitochondrial function in adults is crucial, as these organelles are central to maintaining overall health, influencing everything from energy metabolism to aging and disease. In this exploration, we delve into the intricate world of mitochondria and how their function evolves over the course of adulthood.

Mitochondria: The Cellular Powerhouses

Mitochondria are double-membraned organelles found in the cytoplasm of eukaryotic cells. One of their primary functions is to generate adenosine triphosphate (ATP), the currency of cellular energy. This process, known as oxidative phosphorylation, occurs within the inner mitochondrial membrane and involves a series of complex biochemical reactions.

1. Energy Production:

Mitochondria generate ATP through the electron transport chain (ETC), a sequence of protein complexes embedded in the inner mitochondrial membrane. As electrons move through the ETC, protons are pumped across the membrane, creating a proton gradient. The flow of protons back into the mitochondrial matrix through ATP synthase harnesses the energy to produce ATP.

2. Metabolism and Beyond:

Beyond energy production, mitochondria are intricately involved in metabolic processes.

They regulate fatty acid metabolism, participate in the citric acid cycle (Krebs cycle), and play a role in amino acid metabolism. Additionally, mitochondria are key players in calcium homeostasis, apoptosis (programmed cell death), and the generation of reactive oxygen species (ROS).

Age-Related Changes in Mitochondrial Function:

As adults age, the functional dynamics of mitochondria undergo subtle yet significant changes. These alterations contribute to the aging process and are associated with various age-related diseases. Some key aspects of age-related changes in mitochondrial function include:

1. Decline in ATP Production:

The efficiency of the electron transport chain diminishes with age, leading to a decline in

ATP production. This reduced energy output can impact the overall function of cells, particularly those with high energy demands, such as muscle cells and neurons.

2. Increased Reactive Oxygen Species (ROS) Production:

Aging mitochondria tend to produce more ROS as a byproduct of the electron transport chain. While ROS play a role in signaling and cellular defense mechanisms, an excess can lead to oxidative stress, damaging cellular components and contributing to age-related diseases.

3. Impaired Mitochondrial Dynamics:

Mitochondria are dynamic organelles that undergo fusion and fission, processes essential for maintaining a healthy mitochondrial population. With age, these dynamics can be disrupted, leading to an accumulation of damaged mitochondria and compromised cellular function.

4. Altered Mitochondrial DNA (mtDNA):

Mitochondria have their own DNA (mtDNA), separate from nuclear DNA. The integrity of mtDNA is crucial for mitochondrial function. Over time, mtDNA can accumulate mutations, impairing mitochondrial function and contributing to age-related decline.

Mitochondrial Dysfunction and Disease:

The impact of mitochondrial dysfunction extends beyond the aging process, influencing the development of various diseases in adults.

1. Neurodegenerative Diseases:

Mitochondrial dysfunction is implicated in neurodegenerative disorders such as Alzheimer's, Parkinson's, and Huntington's diseases. Impaired energy production and increased oxidative stress contribute to neuronal damage and cell death.

2. Metabolic Disorders:

Mitochondrial dysfunction is associated with metabolic disorders like diabetes and obesity. Impaired mitochondrial function in insulin-responsive tissues affects glucose metabolism, contributing to insulin resistance.

3. Cardiovascular Diseases:

Mitochondrial dysfunction plays a role in cardiovascular diseases, including heart failure and ischemic heart disease. Insufficient energy production in cardiac muscle cells can compromise the heart's pumping capacity.

4. Aging and Cellular Senescence:

Mitochondrial dysfunction is considered a hallmark of aging. It contributes to cellular senescence, a state where cells lose their ability to divide and function properly. This process is closely linked to age-related diseases.

Strategies to Support Mitochondrial Function:

Given the central role of mitochondria in cellular health, strategies to support their function have gained attention. These include lifestyle interventions and emerging therapeutic approaches.

1. Exercise:

Regular physical activity has been shown to enhance mitochondrial function. Exercise stimulates mitochondrial biogenesis (the creation of new mitochondria), improves mitochondrial dynamics, and enhances oxidative capacity.

2. Nutritional Support:

Certain nutrients play a role in mitochondrial function. Coenzyme Q10, l-carnitine, and antioxidants like vitamin E and C have been studied for their potential to support mitochondrial health.

3. Caloric Restriction:

Caloric restriction, without malnutrition, has been associated with improved mitochondrial function and increased longevity. It may enhance mitochondrial efficiency and reduce oxidative stress.

4. Mitochondrial Targeted Therapies:

Emerging therapeutic approaches focus on directly targeting mitochondria to enhance their function. This includes compounds that stimulate mitochondrial biogenesis or act as antioxidants specifically targeted to mitochondria.

Mitochondrial function is a cornerstone of cellular health, and its impact on adults is profound. As we unravel the intricate details of age-related changes in mitochondrial dynamics, a clearer understanding emerges of their role in health and disease. By exploring strategies to support mitochondrial function, we open avenues for potential interventions that could influence not only the aging process but also the development and progression of various diseases. The ongoing research in this field holds promise for novel therapeutic approaches aimed at preserving and enhancing mitochondrial function, ultimately contributing to healthier and more resilient aging in adults.

Chapter 10: Gene Expression and Adult Health: Decoding the Blueprint of Well-being

Gene expression, the intricate process by which information encoded in our genes is translated into functional molecules within cells, plays a fundamental role in shaping adult health. This complex orchestration of genetic activity influences everything from the development of tissues to the response to environmental factors. In this exploration, we delve into the world of gene expression and its profound impact on the health and well-being of adults.

Gene Expression Basics:

At the core of gene expression is the information transfer from DNA to RNA to proteins. This process involves several key steps:

1. **Transcription:** The first step is transcription, where a specific gene's DNA sequence is transcribed into a complementary RNA molecule. This RNA, known as messenger RNA (mRNA), carries the genetic code from the nucleus to the cytoplasm.

2. **Translation:** In the cytoplasm, the mRNA code is translated into a sequence of amino acids, forming a protein. This is a crucial step as proteins are the functional molecules that carry out most cellular activities.

3. **Regulation:** Gene expression is tightly regulated, and various mechanisms control when and how genes are turned on or off. This regulation is vital for maintaining cellular function, responding to

environmental cues, and adapting to changing conditions.

Epigenetics: Shaping Gene Expression:

Epigenetics adds another layer of complexity to gene expression. It involves modifications to the DNA molecule or associated proteins that can influence gene activity without altering the underlying DNA sequence. Epigenetic modifications play a significant role in determining which genes are active and contribute to the diversity of cell types within the body.

1. **DNA Methylation:** Addition of methyl groups to DNA can repress gene expression. Hypermethylation of certain genes is associated with silencing their activity, impacting cellular functions.

2. **Histone Modifications:** Proteins called histones package DNA into a compact

structure. Modifications to histones can affect the accessibility of genes, influencing whether they are turned on or off.

3. **Non-coding RNAs:** Small RNA molecules, such as microRNAs, can bind to mRNA and prevent translation or promote its degradation, thereby regulating gene expression.

Influence of Gene Expression on Adult Health:

Gene expression is a dynamic process influenced by genetic factors, environmental exposures, and lifestyle choices. Here's how it shapes adult health:

1. Cellular Function and Tissue Development:

Proper gene expression is crucial for the normal development and function of tissues and organs. During adulthood, gene expression ensures the maintenance and repair of tissues, contributing to overall health.

2. Immune System Regulation:

Genes play a central role in regulating the immune system. The expression of specific genes determines the types of immune cells produced, their activation states, and their responses to pathogens. Dysregulation of immune-related genes can contribute to autoimmune diseases or impaired immune function.

3. Metabolic Health:

Gene expression influences metabolic processes, including the regulation of insulin sensitivity, glucose metabolism, and lipid metabolism. Disruptions in gene expression related to metabolism can contribute to conditions such as diabetes and obesity.

4. Response to Environmental Factors:

Gene expression is responsive to environmental factors such as diet, pollutants, and stress. This adaptability allows the body to respond to changing conditions. However, chronic exposure to adverse environments can lead to sustained changes in gene expression that may contribute to disease.

5. Hormonal Regulation:

Hormones act as signaling molecules that regulate gene expression. Hormonal fluctuations during adulthood, such as those associated with the menstrual cycle or aging, can impact gene expression and contribute to physiological changes.

Gene Expression and Aging:

The aging process is intricately linked to changes in gene expression. While genetic factors play a role in determining lifespan and susceptibility to age-related diseases, the dynamic nature of gene expression allows for adaptation and response to aging-related challenges.

1. Senescence and Telomere Shortening: Gene expression is involved in cellular senescence, a state in which cells cease to divide. Telomere shortening, a hallmark of aging, influences gene expression patterns associated with senescence.

2. Mitochondrial Dysfunction: Age-related changes in gene expression contribute to mitochondrial dysfunction, impacting cellular energy production and increasing oxidative stress.

3.   **Inflammation   and   Immune Senescence:** Changes in gene expression contribute to chronic inflammation and immune senescence, both associated with aging and age-related diseases.

Lifestyle and Environmental Influences on Gene Expression:

While genetics provides the blueprint, lifestyle and environmental factors play a crucial role in shaping gene expression throughout adulthood.

1. Diet and Nutrition: Nutrient intake influences gene expression related to metabolism, inflammation, and cellular repair. Certain compounds in foods can also affect epigenetic modifications.

2. Physical Activity: Regular exercise has been shown to influence gene expression patterns associated with cardiovascular health, metabolism, and immune function.

3. Stress and Mental Health: Chronic stress can impact gene expression related to the stress response and inflammation.

Mental health conditions may also be associated with changes in gene expression.

4. Environmental Exposures: Exposure to pollutants, chemicals, and other environmental factors can induce changes in gene expression that may contribute to various health conditions.

Precision Medicine and Gene Expression:

The field of precision medicine aims to tailor medical interventions to individual characteristics, including genetic and epigenetic profiles. Understanding a person's unique gene expression patterns could inform personalized treatment strategies.

1. Cancer Treatment: Precision medicine in cancer often involves analyzing the gene expression profile of tumors to identify specific molecular targets for therapy.

2. Pharmacogenomics: Gene expression patterns can influence how individuals respond to medications. Pharmacogenomic approaches consider genetic and expression variations to optimize drug efficacy and minimize side effects.

3. Disease Risk Prediction: By analyzing gene expression patterns, researchers aim to identify biomarkers that could predict an individual's risk for certain diseases, allowing for early intervention and prevention.

Challenges and Future Directions:

Despite significant progress, challenges persist in fully understanding the complexities of gene expression and its implications for adult health.

1. Interconnected Networks: Genes do not act in isolation but are part of complex networks. Understanding the interplay between genes and how disruptions in one area can affect the entire system poses a challenge.

2. Environmental Variability: The influence of environmental factors on gene expression is vast and variable. Untangling the specific contributions of different factors remains a complex task.

3. Ethical Considerations: The ability to manipulate gene expression raises ethical considerations, particularly in the context of genetic editing and interventions.

4. Longitudinal Studies: Comprehensive longitudinal studies are essential to capture the dynamic changes in gene expression over the course of adulthood, considering the influence of genetics, environment, and lifestyle factors.

In conclusion, gene expression is a dynamic and multifaceted process that profoundly influences adult health. From regulating basic cellular functions to responding to environmental cues, the intricate dance of gene expression shapes our well-being throughout adulthood. As research advances, the integration of genetic, epigenetic, and environmental information holds the promise of a more personalized and precise approach to healthcare, ushering in an era where understanding the language of our genes becomes instrumental in optimizing health and preventing disease.

Chapter 11.1 Cardiovascular Benefits of Hydrogen Medicine for Adults:

Scientific exploration into the cardiovascular benefits of hydrogen medicine for adults has unveiled promising findings that suggest a potential role in maintaining heart health and preventing cardiovascular diseases. Research in this domain has primarily focused on the antioxidant and anti-inflammatory properties of molecular hydrogen and its impact on various cardiovascular parameters.

1. Antioxidant Action:
Numerous studies have highlighted the antioxidant effects of molecular hydrogen. Oxidative stress is a key contributor to cardiovascular diseases, and hydrogen's ability to selectively neutralize harmful reactive oxygen species (ROS) holds

significant therapeutic potential. By reducing oxidative stress, hydrogen may protect vascular endothelial cells and mitigate damage to the cardiovascular system.

2. Anti-Inflammatory Effects:
Chronic inflammation is a hallmark of cardiovascular diseases. Hydrogen has demonstrated anti-inflammatory properties by modulating signaling pathways and reducing the production of pro-inflammatory cytokines. This anti-inflammatory action may contribute to the prevention of atherosclerosis, a condition characterized by inflammation in arterial walls.

3. Blood Pressure Regulation:
Hypertension is a major risk factor for cardiovascular diseases. Studies exploring the effects of hydrogen-rich water or hydrogen gas on blood pressure regulation have reported positive outcomes. Hydrogen's potential to improve endothelial function and modulate blood vessel tone

suggests a role in managing hypertension and promoting vascular health.

4. Improvement in Lipid Profiles:
Dyslipidemia, characterized by abnormal lipid levels, is associated with an increased risk of cardiovascular diseases. Research suggests that hydrogen-rich water may positively influence lipid metabolism, leading to improvements in lipid profiles. This effect could contribute to reducing the risk of atherosclerosis and related cardiovascular events.

5. Protection Against Ischemia-Reperfusion Injury:
Ischemia-reperfusion injury occurs when blood supply is temporarily interrupted and then restored, leading to tissue damage. Hydrogen has demonstrated protective effects against ischemia-reperfusion injury, particularly in the context of myocardial infarction. This suggests a potential

application in preserving heart function during episodes of reduced blood flow.

6. Endothelial Function Enhancement:
The endothelium, the inner lining of blood vessels, plays a crucial role in vascular health. Studies have shown that hydrogen can improve endothelial function, promoting vasodilation and maintaining proper blood flow. Enhanced endothelial function contributes to overall cardiovascular well-being.

7. Reduction in Myocardial Injury Markers:
Hydrogen's ability to reduce markers of myocardial injury, such as troponin and creatine kinase, has been observed in experimental studies. These findings imply a protective effect on cardiac tissue and suggest potential applications in preventing or mitigating damage following cardiac events.

8. Clinical Trials and Translational Research:

While many preclinical studies have provided insights into the cardiovascular benefits of hydrogen, ongoing clinical trials aim to validate these findings in human populations. Translational research is essential for bridging the gap between laboratory discoveries and practical applications in clinical settings.

In summary, the scientific studies on hydrogen medicine for cardiovascular health in adults underscore its potential as a therapeutic intervention. The antioxidant, anti-inflammatory, and vascular protective effects of molecular hydrogen present a compelling case for further exploration, with implications for preventing and managing cardiovascular diseases.

11.2 Neurological Effects of Hydrogen Medicine for Adults:

The burgeoning field of hydrogen medicine has extended its reach into the realm of neurological health, with studies suggesting a range of potential benefits for adults. The neurological effects of molecular hydrogen have been investigated in various contexts, including neuroprotection, cognitive function, and the management of neurodegenerative disorders.

1. Neuroprotective Properties:

Molecular hydrogen has demonstrated neuroprotective effects in preclinical studies. Its ability to act as an antioxidant and reduce oxidative stress is particularly relevant in the context of neurodegenerative diseases where oxidative damage plays a significant role. By scavenging reactive oxygen species (ROS), hydrogen may help preserve neuronal integrity and function.

2. Mitigation of Inflammation in the Brain:

Chronic neuroinflammation is a common feature of several neurological disorders. Hydrogen exhibits anti-inflammatory properties, modulating inflammatory pathways and reducing the production of pro-inflammatory cytokines. This anti-inflammatory action may contribute to mitigating inflammation in the brain and potentially slowing the progression of neurodegenerative conditions.

3. Impact on Cognitive Function:

Cognitive decline is a concern in aging adults, and hydrogen's effects on cognitive function have been explored. Studies suggest that hydrogen may have cognitive-enhancing properties, possibly linked to its ability to protect against oxidative stress and support overall brain health. These findings open avenues for investigating hydrogen as a potential intervention for age-related cognitive decline.

4. Potential in Stroke Rehabilitation:
Ischemic stroke results in damage to brain tissue due to reduced blood flow. Hydrogen has shown promise in preclinical models for its ability to reduce oxidative stress and inflammation in the aftermath of a stroke. This suggests a potential role in stroke rehabilitation and recovery.

5. Alleviation of Parkinson's and Alzheimer's Symptoms:
Hydrogen has been investigated for its potential therapeutic effects in Parkinson's and Alzheimer's diseases. Preclinical studies suggest that hydrogen may alleviate symptoms associated with these neurodegenerative disorders, providing a novel approach for managing these challenging conditions.

6. Modulation of Neurotransmitter Systems:

Hydrogen has been shown to modulate neurotransmitter systems, including glutamate and gamma-aminobutyric acid (GABA). These effects on neurotransmission could have implications for conditions characterized by imbalances in neurotransmitter levels.

7. Brain Edema and Traumatic Brain Injury:

Studies have explored the role of hydrogen in reducing brain edema and mitigating damage in traumatic brain injury (TBI). Hydrogen's anti-inflammatory and antioxidant properties may contribute to limiting secondary injury processes in the aftermath of TBI.

8. Clinical Trials and Translation to Human Studies:

While the preclinical evidence is promising, the translation of these findings into clinical applications is a critical step. Ongoing and future clinical trials will provide valuable insights into the safety and efficacy of hydrogen therapy for neurological conditions in human populations.

In conclusion, the scientific exploration of hydrogen medicine's neurological effects in adults offers a compelling narrative of potential therapeutic benefits. From neuroprotection to cognitive enhancement and the management of neurodegenerative disorders, hydrogen's multifaceted actions on the central nervous system warrant continued investigation for their translational potential.

11.3 Anti-Cancer Potential of Hydrogen Medicine for Adults:

The investigation into the potential anti-cancer effects of hydrogen medicine in adults represents a fascinating frontier in medical research. While the field is relatively young, preclinical studies have provided intriguing insights into the ability of molecular hydrogen to influence various aspects of cancer development and progression.

1. Antioxidant and Anti-Inflammatory Actions:

Hydrogen's fundamental properties as an antioxidant and anti-inflammatory agent form the basis of its potential anti-cancer effects. By reducing oxidative stress and inflammation, hydrogen may help create an environment less conducive to cancer initiation and progression.

2. DNA Protection and Repair:

Hydrogen's impact on DNA integrity is a crucial aspect of its anti-cancer potential. Studies have suggested that hydrogen may protect against DNA damage induced by reactive oxygen species (ROS) and enhance DNA repair mechanisms. Preserving the stability of the genome is a key factor in preventing cancer development.

3. Apoptosis Induction in Cancer Cells:

Apoptosis, or programmed cell death, is a natural process that helps regulate cell populations and eliminate damaged cells. Hydrogen has shown promise in inducing apoptosis specifically in cancer cells while sparing normal cells. This selective action is crucial for developing targeted and less harmful cancer therapies.

4. Inhibition of Angiogenesis:

Angiogenesis, the formation of new blood vessels, is a process essential for tumor growth and metastasis. Hydrogen has been investigated for its potential to inhibit angiogenesis, thereby restricting the blood supply to tumors. By impeding this process, hydrogen may interfere with cancer progression.

5. Enhanced Sensitivity to Cancer Treatments:

Preclinical studies suggest that hydrogen may enhance the sensitivity of cancer cells to conventional treatments such as chemotherapy and radiation therapy. This synergistic effect could potentially improve the efficacy of standard cancer treatments while minimizing side effects.

6. Reduction in Metastatic Potential:

Metastasis, the spread of cancer cells to distant organs, is a major challenge in cancer management. Hydrogen has shown promise in reducing the metastatic potential of cancer cells, potentially limiting the spread of the disease to other parts of the body.

7. Modulation of Immune Responses:
The immune system plays a crucial role in surveilling and eliminating cancer cells. Hydrogen has been investigated for its immunomodulatory effects, including the enhancement of natural killer (NK) cell activity and other immune responses. This modulation may contribute to the body's ability to recognize and eliminate cancer cells.

8. Effects on Cancer Stem Cells:
Cancer stem cells are a subset of cells within tumors with the ability to self-renew and contribute to tumor growth. Studies have explored the impact of hydrogen on cancer stem cells, with some suggesting inhibitory effects. Targeting these cells is critical for preventing cancer recurrence.

9. Reduction in Treatment-Induced Side Effects:

In addition to its potential anti-cancer effects, hydrogen has been investigated for its ability to reduce side effects associated with cancer treatments. This includes mitigating radiation-induced damage to normal tissues and minimizing chemotherapy-related toxicity.

10. Clinical Trials and Translation to Human Applications:

While the preclinical evidence is promising, the transition to clinical trials is a crucial step in determining the safety and efficacy of hydrogen therapy for cancer in human populations. Ongoing and future trials will provide valuable insights into its potential role as an adjuvant therapy or standalone treatment.

In summary, the anti-cancer potential of hydrogen medicine for adults is a compelling area of research with diverse implications for cancer prevention and treatment. From influencing fundamental cellular processes to enhancing treatment responses and reducing side effects, the multifaceted actions of molecular hydrogen open new avenues for innovative approaches to cancer care.

11.4 Metabolic Health in Adults and Hydrogen Medicine:

The interplay between hydrogen medicine and metabolic health in adults has become a subject of increasing interest in scientific research. Metabolic health encompasses various factors, including glucose regulation, lipid metabolism, and overall energy balance. Here, we explore the evolving landscape of studies investigating the impact of hydrogen on metabolic health in adults.

1. Glucose Metabolism and Insulin Sensitivity:

Preclinical studies have suggested that hydrogen may have beneficial effects on glucose metabolism and insulin sensitivity. Hydrogen-rich water has been shown to improve insulin resistance, potentially contributing to better blood glucose control. This holds significance for individuals with metabolic disorders, such as type 2 diabetes.

2. Lipid Profiles and Cardiovascular Risk:

Dyslipidemia, characterized by abnormal lipid levels, is a key factor in cardiovascular risk. Hydrogen has shown promise in modulating lipid profiles, including reducing levels of total cholesterol and low-density lipoprotein (LDL) cholesterol. These lipid-lowering effects may contribute to the prevention of atherosclerosis and cardiovascular diseases.

3. Weight Management and Adiposity:

Obesity is a major risk factor for metabolic disorders, and studies have explored the potential role of hydrogen in weight management. While the evidence is preliminary, some research suggests that hydrogen may influence adiposity and contribute to maintaining a healthy body weight.

4. Mitochondrial Function and Energy Balance:

Mitochondria play a central role in energy production and metabolic regulation. Hydrogen's interactions with mitochondria have been studied for their potential impact on energy balance. By enhancing mitochondrial function, hydrogen may contribute to overall metabolic health.

5. Inflammation and Metabolic Syndrome:

Chronic inflammation is closely linked to metabolic syndrome, a cluster of conditions that increase the risk of heart disease, stroke, and type 2 diabetes. Hydrogen's anti-inflammatory properties may have implications for managing inflammation associated with metabolic syndrome.

6. Oxidative Stress and Cellular Metabolism:

The relationship between oxidative stress and metabolic health is intricate. Hydrogen's role as an antioxidant may help counteract oxidative stress associated with metabolic imbalances, potentially influencing cellular metabolism in a favorable manner.

7. Regulation of Appetite and Food Intake:

Some studies have explored the impact of hydrogen on appetite regulation and food intake. While the mechanisms are not fully understood, there are indications that hydrogen may influence factors related to satiety and eating behavior.

8. Exercise Performance and Recovery:
Metabolic health extends to physical performance, and hydrogen has been investigated for its potential effects on exercise performance and recovery. Studies suggest that hydrogen may have anti-fatigue properties and could enhance exercise-induced improvements in metabolic parameters.

9. Clinical Applications and Human Trials:
Translating the preclinical findings into clinical applications is a crucial step in determining the real-world impact of hydrogen on metabolic health. Clinical trials are underway to investigate the safety and efficacy of hydrogen therapy in adults with metabolic disorders.

10. Overall Impact on Healthspan:

Metabolic health is intricately connected to overall well-being and the aging process. Research into hydrogen's effects on metabolic parameters contributes to the broader concept of healthspan—the length of time an individual remains in good health.

In conclusion, the scientific studies on hydrogen medicine and metabolic health in adults underscore the potential for hydrogen to influence key aspects of metabolism, from glucose regulation to lipid metabolism. While research is ongoing, the findings suggest a nuanced interplay between hydrogen and metabolic processes, opening avenues for innovative approaches to metabolic disorders and overall health.

Chapter 12: Clinical Applications of Hydrogen Medicine for Adult Patients: Unraveling Therapeutic Potential

The clinical applications of hydrogen medicine for adult patients have been gaining traction, with research shedding light on its diverse therapeutic potential across various medical conditions. From its antioxidant properties to anti-inflammatory effects, hydrogen has emerged as a promising intervention in both preventive and therapeutic healthcare strategies. In this exploration, we delve into the clinical applications of hydrogen medicine and its potential impact on adult patients across a spectrum of health challenges.

1. Cardiovascular Health:

Hydrogen's cardiovascular benefits extend into clinical applications for adult patients dealing with heart-related conditions. Studies have explored its potential in managing hypertension, reducing oxidative stress, and improving endothelial function. Clinical trials are underway to investigate the efficacy of hydrogen therapy in reducing the risk of cardiovascular events and improving overall heart health. As a complementary approach, hydrogen-rich water or gas could become part of interventions aimed at preventing or managing cardiovascular diseases, such as atherosclerosis and heart failure.

2. Neurological Disorders:

Clinical applications of hydrogen medicine in neurological disorders hold promise for conditions like Alzheimer's, Parkinson's, and ischemic stroke. Hydrogen's neuroprotective properties, including its ability to mitigate oxidative stress and inflammation, make it a compelling candidate for interventions targeting neurodegenerative diseases. Ongoing clinical trials are exploring the safety and efficacy of hydrogen therapy in improving cognitive function, reducing neuroinflammation, and potentially slowing the progression of neurodegenerative disorders in adult patients.

3. Cancer Treatment Support:

In the realm of oncology, hydrogen medicine is being investigated for its potential as an adjuvant therapy. Clinical applications include utilizing hydrogen-rich solutions alongside conventional cancer treatments like chemotherapy and radiation therapy. Research suggests that hydrogen may enhance the sensitivity of cancer cells to treatment, reduce side effects, and potentially improve the overall efficacy of cancer therapies. Clinical trials aim to validate these findings and establish hydrogen therapy as a safe and effective supportive measure in cancer care for adult patients.

4. Metabolic Disorders:

The clinical applications of hydrogen medicine in metabolic disorders, such as type 2 diabetes and obesity, are being explored with increasing interest. Studies suggest that hydrogen may positively influence glucose metabolism, insulin sensitivity, and lipid profiles. This opens avenues for hydrogen therapy as an adjunct to standard treatments, potentially contributing to better glycemic control and metabolic health in adult patients. Clinical trials are crucial for determining the feasibility and effectiveness of incorporating hydrogen-rich solutions into the management of metabolic disorders.

5. Gastrointestinal Health:

Hydrogen's anti-inflammatory and antioxidant properties have implications for gastrointestinal health, making it a subject of interest in conditions like inflammatory bowel disease (IBD) and irritable bowel syndrome (IBS). Clinical applications include exploring the potential of hydrogen therapy to reduce inflammation, alleviate symptoms, and contribute to the overall well-being of adult patients dealing with gastrointestinal challenges. Clinical trials are essential for elucidating the therapeutic impact of hydrogen-rich solutions in gastrointestinal disorders.

6. Respiratory Conditions:

The therapeutic potential of hydrogen medicine extends to respiratory conditions, including chronic obstructive pulmonary disease (COPD) and asthma. Hydrogen's anti-inflammatory effects may play a role in mitigating airway inflammation and improving respiratory function. Clinical applications involve investigating hydrogen therapy as a complementary approach to conventional treatments, with a focus on alleviating symptoms and enhancing the quality of life for adult patients with respiratory disorders.

7. Skin Health and Dermatological Conditions:

Hydrogen's role in skin health and dermatological conditions is an emerging area of clinical exploration. Preliminary studies suggest that hydrogen may have antioxidant and anti-inflammatory effects beneficial for conditions like dermatitis and wound healing. Clinical applications involve assessing the potential of hydrogen-rich solutions in dermatological interventions, offering a novel approach to supporting skin health in adult patients.

8. Anti-Aging Interventions:

The potential anti-aging effects of hydrogen medicine are a subject of interest in clinical applications. Hydrogen's impact on oxidative stress, mitochondrial function, and cellular senescence make it a candidate for interventions aimed at promoting healthy aging. Clinical trials are underway to investigate the feasibility of incorporating hydrogen therapy into anti-aging protocols, potentially influencing healthspan and overall well-being in adult patients.

9. Postoperative Recovery:

Hydrogen's ability to mitigate oxidative stress and inflammation has implications for postoperative recovery. Clinical applications include exploring hydrogen therapy as a supportive measure for surgical patients, aiming to enhance recovery, reduce inflammation, and minimize complications. Clinical trials are crucial for establishing the safety and efficacy of incorporating hydrogen-rich solutions into postoperative care protocols for adult patients.

10. Psychological Well-being:

The potential impact of hydrogen medicine on psychological well-being is an area of growing interest. Research suggests that hydrogen may have neuroprotective and mood-modulating effects. Clinical applications involve exploring hydrogen therapy as a supportive measure in mental health interventions, potentially contributing to stress reduction and overall psychological well-being in adult patients.

Challenges and Future Directions:

While the clinical applications of hydrogen medicine hold promise, several challenges and questions remain. The optimal dosages, delivery methods, and long-term safety profiles need further investigation. Standardization of protocols and the identification of specific patient populations that may benefit the most are essential for the widespread acceptance of hydrogen therapy in clinical settings.

Hydrogen medicine's journey from laboratory discoveries to clinical applications is a dynamic and evolving process. The diverse therapeutic potential observed in preclinical studies has prompted an array of clinical trials across various medical disciplines. As the research landscape expands, the hope is that hydrogen medicine will find its place as a complementary and innovative approach to improving health outcomes for adult patients facing a range of conditions. The ongoing collaboration between researchers, clinicians, and patients is vital for unraveling the full clinical potential of hydrogen medicine and translating it into effective and evidence-based healthcare interventions.

Chapter 13: Safety Considerations in Adult Hydrogen Therapy: Navigating the Path to Wellness

Hydrogen therapy, harnessing the potential health benefits of molecular hydrogen, has emerged as a subject of significant scientific interest and clinical exploration. As researchers and healthcare practitioners delve into the potential therapeutic applications of hydrogen for adults, it is imperative to prioritize safety considerations. This comprehensive review examines the safety aspects of hydrogen therapy, addressing concerns, highlighting key findings, and exploring the path forward in ensuring the well-being of individuals undergoing hydrogen-based interventions.

1. Inhalation vs. Ingestion vs. Topical Application:

Hydrogen therapy can be administered through various methods, including inhalation, ingestion (via hydrogen-rich water or hydrogen-infused beverages), and topical application. Each route comes with its safety considerations. Inhalation requires careful monitoring of gas concentrations to prevent potential risks, while ingestion may involve assessing the quality and purity of hydrogen-infused products. Topical application, such as hydrogen-rich baths, necessitates attention to factors like water temperature and exposure duration.

2. Gas Concentrations and Inhalation Safety:

Inhalation of hydrogen gas is one of the primary methods of administration in clinical settings. Safety considerations revolve around determining optimal gas concentrations that provide therapeutic benefits without posing risks. High concentrations of hydrogen may have an anesthetic effect, emphasizing the importance of precise control over gas levels during inhalation therapy to avoid adverse reactions.

3. Potential Flammability and Explosion Risks:

Hydrogen is flammable, and safety protocols must be in place to mitigate potential risks. Adequate ventilation, explosion-proof equipment, and adherence to established safety guidelines are crucial, particularly in settings where hydrogen gas is generated or administered. Rigorous safety measures are essential to prevent accidents and ensure the secure use of hydrogen-based therapies.

4. Hydrogen Purity and Contamination:

The purity of the hydrogen used in therapy is paramount. Impurities, even in trace amounts, can compromise the safety and efficacy of hydrogen interventions. Quality control measures during the production and administration of hydrogen are essential to minimize the risk of unintended reactions or side effects associated with impurities.

5. Individual Variability and Health Status:

Safety considerations in hydrogen therapy extend to individual variability in response and health status. Factors such as age, pre-existing medical conditions, and medications can influence how individuals respond to hydrogen. Comprehensive health assessments and personalized treatment plans, guided by healthcare professionals, are crucial to ensuring the safety of adult patients undergoing hydrogen therapy.

6. Duration and Frequency of Administration:

The optimal duration and frequency of hydrogen therapy sessions are areas of ongoing research and safety considerations. While hydrogen has shown therapeutic potential, determining the most effective and safe treatment regimens requires careful examination. Balancing the desire for therapeutic benefits with a cautious approach to prevent overexposure or excessive treatment durations is essential.

7. Long-Term Safety and Chronic Exposure:

Long-term safety considerations are paramount, especially as hydrogen therapy gains popularity as a potential intervention for chronic conditions. Limited data exist on the effects of prolonged exposure to hydrogen, emphasizing the need for longitudinal studies to assess the safety profile of extended hydrogen therapy in adults. Understanding the potential cumulative effects over time is crucial for establishing the safety of chronic hydrogen exposure.

8. Potential Interactions with Medications:

As with any therapeutic intervention, potential interactions between hydrogen therapy and medications must be carefully considered. Hydrogen's influence on cellular and molecular processes may interact with pharmacological agents, impacting drug metabolism or efficacy. Close collaboration between healthcare providers and patients is essential to evaluate potential interactions and adjust treatment plans accordingly.

9. Adverse Effects and Reporting Mechanisms:

Monitoring and reporting adverse effects are integral components of ensuring safety in hydrogen therapy. The identification and documentation of any unexpected reactions or side effects contribute to a comprehensive understanding of the therapy's safety profile. Establishing clear reporting mechanisms and communication channels between healthcare professionals, researchers, and patients is crucial for ongoing safety assessment.

10. Precautions for Vulnerable Populations:

Certain populations, such as pregnant individuals, individuals with respiratory conditions, and those with compromised health, may require specific precautions when undergoing hydrogen therapy. Research on the safety and efficacy of hydrogen interventions in vulnerable populations is limited, necessitating a cautious approach and tailored safety protocols.

11. Regulatory Oversight and Guidelines:

The establishment of regulatory oversight and guidelines for hydrogen therapy is an evolving process. Authorities need to play a proactive role in defining safety standards, monitoring therapeutic interventions, and providing clear guidelines for practitioners. Collaboration between researchers, clinicians, and regulatory bodies is essential for creating a framework that ensures the safe and responsible use of hydrogen therapy.

12. Education and Informed Consent:

Ensuring safety in hydrogen therapy involves comprehensive education and informed consent processes for individuals undergoing such interventions. Patients should receive detailed information about the potential risks, benefits, and uncertainties associated with hydrogen therapy. Informed consent allows individuals to make autonomous decisions regarding their participation in hydrogen-based interventions while understanding the potential safety considerations.

Conclusion and Future Directions:

As the field of hydrogen therapy continues to advance, a proactive approach to safety considerations is paramount. Rigorous research, adherence to safety protocols, and ongoing monitoring of adverse effects are essential components of ensuring the well-being of adult patients undergoing hydrogen-based interventions. Future directions should prioritize the establishment of standardized safety guidelines, long-term safety assessments, and regulatory frameworks to foster responsible and evidence-based use of hydrogen therapy in diverse healthcare settings. Through collaborative efforts, the scientific and medical communities can navigate the path to wellness, harnessing the therapeutic potential of hydrogen while prioritizing the safety of those seeking its benefits.

Chapter 14: Conclusion: Integrating Hydrogen Medicine into Adult Healthcare - A Paradigm Shift in Wellness

The exploration of hydrogen medicine, with its potential therapeutic applications, has unfolded a new chapter in adult healthcare. As the scientific community delves into the multifaceted benefits of molecular hydrogen, there is growing anticipation surrounding its integration into mainstream healthcare practices. In this comprehensive conclusion, we reflect on the journey of hydrogen medicine, its diverse applications, and the transformative impact it could have on adult healthcare.

1. The Evolution of Hydrogen Medicine:

Hydrogen, once overlooked as a simple diatomic gas, has transitioned from a background player to a potential protagonist in the realm of healthcare. The journey began with the recognition of hydrogen's antioxidant properties and its ability to selectively neutralize harmful free radicals. From there, research expanded to unravel its anti-inflammatory effects, neuroprotective qualities, and potential in addressing a spectrum of health conditions.

2. Diverse Therapeutic Applications:

The versatility of hydrogen's therapeutic applications has been a defining characteristic of its journey in adult healthcare. From cardiovascular health to neurological disorders, cancer treatment support, metabolic disorders, and beyond, hydrogen has shown promise in influencing fundamental biological processes. The array of potential applications underscores the complexity of hydrogen's interactions at the cellular and molecular levels.

3. Cardiovascular Benefits and Neuroprotection:

Hydrogen's cardiovascular benefits, including its role in blood pressure regulation, improvement of lipid profiles, and protection against ischemic events, point to its potential as a preventive measure against heart-related conditions. Simultaneously, its neuroprotective effects in mitigating oxidative stress and inflammation offer a new frontier in addressing neurological disorders and promoting cognitive well-being in adults.

4. Oncology and Metabolic Disorders:

The journey of hydrogen medicine extends into the realms of oncology and metabolic health. As a potential adjuvant therapy in cancer treatment, hydrogen's ability to sensitize cancer cells to conventional therapies and reduce treatment-related side effects opens avenues for more holistic and patient-centric approaches. In metabolic disorders, its impact on glucose metabolism, insulin sensitivity, and lipid profiles provides a promising avenue for managing conditions like diabetes and obesity.

5. Safety Considerations and Responsible Integration:

As hydrogen medicine moves closer to widespread integration into adult healthcare, safety considerations remain a focal point. Rigorous research, adherence to safety protocols, and ongoing monitoring of adverse effects are essential components of ensuring the well-being of individuals undergoing hydrogen-based interventions.

The responsible integration of hydrogen therapy requires clear regulatory oversight, standardized guidelines, and continuous collaboration between researchers, healthcare practitioners, and regulatory bodies.

6. Personalized Healthcare and Precision Medicine:

Hydrogen medicine aligns seamlessly with the principles of personalized healthcare and precision medicine. The understanding that individuals respond differently to interventions underscores the importance of tailoring hydrogen therapy to the unique characteristics of each patient. Genetic, epigenetic, and lifestyle factors can influence how hydrogen interacts within the body, emphasizing the need for a nuanced and personalized approach in healthcare delivery.

7. Collaboration Between Research and Clinical Practice:

The successful integration of hydrogen medicine into adult healthcare hinges on a harmonious collaboration between the realms of research and clinical practice. Researchers play a pivotal role in expanding the scientific understanding of hydrogen's mechanisms of action, uncovering new applications, and contributing to the evidence base supporting its therapeutic potential. Healthcare practitioners, in turn, apply this knowledge in real-world settings, translating research findings into effective and personalized interventions for their patients.

8. Challenges and Future Directions:

While the journey of hydrogen medicine has been marked by promising discoveries, challenges and unanswered questions persist. The need for standardized dosages, optimal delivery methods, and long-term safety assessments requires further exploration. The dynamic interplay between genetics, environment, and individual variability presents a complex puzzle that researchers and clinicians aim to decipher. Ongoing efforts to address these challenges will pave the way for a more robust and comprehensive understanding of hydrogen's role in adult healthcare.

9. Holistic Approach to Wellness:

The integration of hydrogen medicine into adult healthcare signifies a broader shift towards a holistic approach to wellness. Recognizing the interconnectedness of biological systems, the potential of hydrogen to influence various aspects of health offers a holistic perspective on preventive and therapeutic interventions. By addressing oxidative stress, inflammation, and cellular dysfunction, hydrogen contributes to a more comprehensive understanding of well-being.

10. Patient Empowerment and Informed Decision-Making:

As hydrogen medicine becomes part of the healthcare landscape, patient empowerment and informed decision-making take center stage. Educating individuals about the potential benefits, risks, and uncertainties associated with hydrogen therapy empowers them to make informed choices aligned with their health goals. Shared decision-making between healthcare providers and patients fosters a collaborative and patient-centric approach to care.

11. The Promise of a Paradigm Shift:

In conclusion, the integration of hydrogen medicine into adult healthcare holds the promise of a paradigm shift in how we approach health and well-being. Beyond traditional interventions, the potential of hydrogen to modulate cellular processes and promote resilience opens new avenues for optimizing health and preventing disease. As research advances, clinical applications expand, and safety considerations are refined, the transformative impact of hydrogen medicine on adult healthcare is poised to reshape the landscape of wellness.

12. The Continuum of Discovery:

The journey of hydrogen medicine is an ongoing continuum of discovery, characterized by the dynamic interplay between research, clinical practice, and the evolving understanding of human biology. As researchers delve deeper into the molecular nuances of hydrogen's actions and clinicians apply these insights in diverse healthcare settings, the potential for groundbreaking discoveries and transformative healthcare solutions remains boundless.

In the grand tapestry of adult healthcare, hydrogen medicine emerges as a vibrant thread, weaving its way through the intricacies of biological systems and offering a new perspective on health optimization.

www.ingramcontent.com/pod-product-compliance
Lightning Source LLC
Chambersburg PA
CBHW071047290526

45795CB00004B/1360